THE STINKEST PARTS OF A WOMAN'S BODY

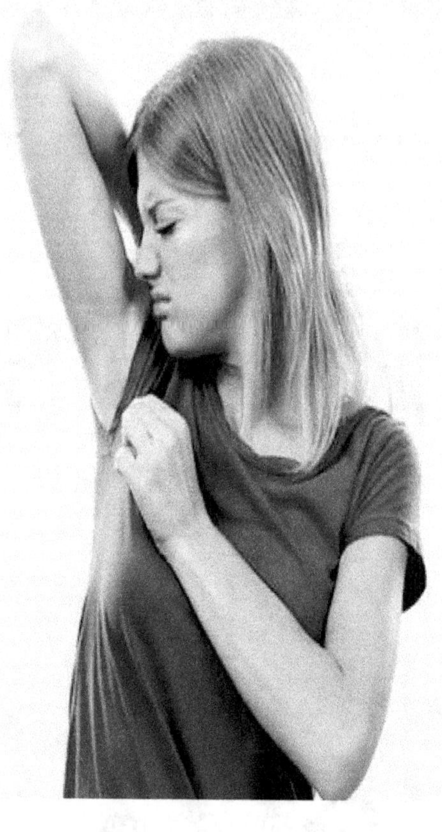

Contents

Copyright © 2017

All rights reserved. No part of this publication may be reproduced, distributed, or transmitted in any form or by any means, including photocopying, recording, or other electronic or mechanical methods, without the prior written permission of the publisher, except in the case of brief quotations embodied in critical reviews certain other noncommercial uses permitted by copyright law

Practicing and maintaining good physical hygiene is crucial to avoiding complications in the woman's' body private areas. As it is, in the western culture, our armpits, feet, anal, vaginal, and pelvic areas are secluded from open fresh air many hours of any given day. These areas have creases in the skin that traps in moisture hastening the probability of bacteria growth if not thoroughly cleansed with mild soap and warm water daily. For some, several times a day. While it is important for men and women to execute healthy hygiene habits, it is even more so for the woman. While some women typically build up an odor in their feet (especially if they have worn socks and encased shoes all day), armpits, and private areas, they have also added probability of obtaining a strong fish like odor in and around her vagina if proper body hygiene is not adhered to daily.

Because the vagina is made up soft, moist tissue, it is not uncommon for a woman to periodically experience a light odor by the end of a day. Often times, this may result in a slight vaginal discharge as well.

Those who live in warmer climates, yet forced by society to cover up for fear of arrest for indecent exposure may experience it even more so. Other lifestyles that may cause a smelly vaginal odor and discharge is that of a dancer, gymnast, deep sea diver, etc.

These sports require the athlete to wear non-breathable fabric such as nylon ballet tights, spandex leotards, and full bodied rubber suits for hours at a time while executing physical exertion adding even more heat to the already creviced and enclosed areas.

Entrapping the vagina and other bodily parts with folds of skin or tissue to trap in the moisture causing bacteria to form and grow. For the woman, this may result in a slight vaginal yeast infection. If left unchecked, it could grow into a health problem.

Women are beautiful creatures. In order for the body scent to reflect the inner and outer beauty of the woman, do not just cover up with perfumes. Take good care of the vessel you have been given. Practice good hygiene and enjoy being a woman.

In this GUIDE, we will explore some stinking parts of the woman's body and ways to overcome those stinking odors.

LET'S GET STARTED!

CHAPTER 1

PERSPIRATION

While others hate sweat and the corresponding body odor (BO) that it brings, women who have been blessed with little perspiration have a lot to be thankful for.

Actually without realizing it, these women probably have more than enough perspiration. We lose about half a liter of water everyday by perspiring without noticing it. This is called insensible perspiration. As the temperature of the body rises, sweat forms on the surface of the skin and evaporates to cool this.

Anidrosis is a condition in which sweat is absent from the body but this usually affects the elderly, those with a thyroid deficiency, and certain skin diseases. Women with anidrosis may collapse from over¬heating after exercising. Symptoms include nausea, dizziness, and dehydration.Most women who don't perspire as much as they think actually do but their sweat evaporates easily. This prevents it from being contaminated with bacteria causing BO.

How does BO start? Fresh sweat is free from odor. Perspiration that evaporates easily cannot offend even the most discriminating nostril. Body odor starts when the evaporation process is hampered by clothing or body folds like the arms, breasts, thighs and the genital area. The offensive odor is the result of bacterial action.

Personal cleanliness is still the best way to prevent BO. Sometimes, a good bath and loose clothes are all that's needed to solve the problem.

Deodorants only mask odors but they will not reduce perspiration like antiperspirants. Creams and roll-ons generally give greater protection but are messier than aerosol products. Wet aerosols, on the other hand, are known to give one a sticky, wet, cold, burning or irritating feeling. If this happens, discontinue using the product.

If you still have BO after bathing, using clean, loose clothes and a good antiperspirant deodorant, you may be suffering from certain diseases. Consult a doctor regarding this matter.

CHAPTER 2

Every woman is susceptible to having offensive feminine odor because this is a condition brought about by several factors. There are a few common causes of feminine odor that can be easily prevented, and there are also some that are difficult to deal with.

The following are the common causes of feminine odor that you should be aware of.

1. Bacterial vaginosis

This happens when the natural balance of micro-organisms in your genital are disrupted, causing the bad bacteria to multiply. Bacterial vaginosis or BV is often associated with green-like or grayish discharge which gives off a fishy smell. This smell is actually the offensive vaginal odor that scares all women.

2. Infection and STD

Yeast infection and sexually transmitted diseases like Chlamydia, Gonorrhea and the like are also major causes of feminine odor. The odor comes from the substance that bacteria carry, and so when bacteria multiply the amount of this offensive odor-causing substance also increases. This turns the foul odor into a severely unpleasant vaginal odor.

3. Bad Hygiene

It is imperative that women should keep their bodies clean, fresh and fragrant because poor hygiene is a major turn off. Not to mention that it can result in bad body odor and unpleasant feminine smell.

Since female's genitalia are prone to acquiring infection due to its physical make-up, it is essential to keep them clean and dry. Otherwise, moisture and other environmental elements may intervene with the natural flow of the vaginal organisms.

4. Retained tampons and sanitary pads

When a woman has period, she is vulnerable to have a distinct kind of feminine odor. This is not because of the menstruation per se, but the accumulated blood in the tampons and sanitary pads. When you have your menstruation, make it a point to change tampons and pads as often as possible.

5. Pelvic Inflammatory Disease (PID), cancer and other chronic disease

If a woman suffers from a terminal disease like pelvic cancer or PID, she is likely to have an offensive feminine odor. This is not easy to manage because of the disease involved, although keeping your genitalia clean will eliminate the smell momentarily.

6. Multiple sex partners

Having more than one sexual partner is one of the causes of feminine odor. The condition can even get worse if you don't practice safe sex.

7. Wearing non-cotton undergarments

Since female's genital area is prone to infection, it needs to stay dry and clean. That is why cotton panty is highly recommended as it keeps the area free from sweat and moisture.

8. Dirty toilet seat and public swimming pools

Sitting on a dirty toilet seat or dipping in to a public swimming pool can cause bacterial invasion to a woman's genital area. This can cause infection that will lead to bad feminine smell.

These causes of feminine odor can be treated either by medication or by natural remedies. In fact, some causes can be resolved by just observing proper hygiene.

CHAPTER 3

THE HAIR

A woman's hair is her crown, and it should always be treated with love and respect. So is the principle of most women all over the world: seldom do we see women with unkempt hair, as most women fix their hair before going out of the house.

This is also why the smallest hair problems bother most of these females. What should be remembered is that good hair is only a result of well-maintained scalp.

Here are a few scalp issues and solutions for better hair maintenance:

Itchiness, Flakes and Dandruff

For itchiness and flakes caused by dandruff, use a moisturizing dandruff shampoo once or twice a week. Do not forget to use products with SPF, as flakes and itchiness may also be caused by sunburn.

Your hair might also be itchy even if you do not have dandruff. This is most likely caused by an abundance of yeast in your body, and not because of dry skin as most people would believe.

To remedy itchy scalp, use products with Tea Tree Oil. Tea Tree Oil is a natural anti-fungal ingredient and is also known to be a scalp stimulant. Shampooing also helps exfoliate dead skin cells from the scalp that can cause build-up and itchiness.

If you wish to go organic and try homemade treatments, make use of apple cider vinegar. It is also one of the most effective ways to keep your mane shiny and lustrous.

To use, rinse your tresses with 1 part apple cider vinegar with 3 parts water after washing. Also, you might want to invest in a good supplement containing acidophilus, as this is also regulates yeast, a great treatment for itchy scalp.

Bad Mane Odor

Smelly hair is the tress equivalent of body odor - no one wants to be caught having one, nor smell one! Like body odor, bad odor in your mane is also caused by lack of cleaning, especially when you don't clean your hair daily.

Like the skin on the body, the skin on the scalp has sweat and oil glands. If unwashed for a few days, the sweat and oil start to build up and the bacteria that naturally are contained in the body starts to break down and cause a stench as it reacts with the air and the oil, and spoils in effect.

This, however, doesn't happen just after a day of not washing your hair, but as it reaches the end of the second to the start of the third day, smells begin to crop up.

Although actually washing your mane everyday with shampoo is not only unrealistic (to some women) but also isn't the best way to go (especially for some women with color-treated hair, as this leads to premature color fading), washing it every other day or every third day is the best alternative to avoid smelly locks.

Women with thicker and coarser locks have less oil glands per square inch due to their thicker individual strands, which makes them less vulnerable to excess grease compared to women with fine tresses, since they have more oil glands per square inch.

If you are like most women who are used to just washing their hair every other day (or every third day), preventing or camouflaging bad hair odors can be done by using dry shampoos, as these products soak up excess oil and gives a fragrance that covers any unwanted smells.

Lastly, preventing or treating these problems isn't just about obtaining great, good-smelling hair, but it is also about keeping your scalp nourished and healthy. Your hair grows best with a healthy environment, regular washing, and proper diet.

CHAPTER 4

THE MOUTH

The human body creates a range of odors in the form of volatile chemical substances that stimulate the sense of smell. It's a natural process that you can't prevent and this is why so many people look for a treatment to rid odors such as bad breath or smelly feet.

All-natural functions of the body serve a purpose which also applies to smell. If it wasn't for certain odors that alert us to dangerous conditions we could die. What makes matters worse is there is no natural odor with a pleasant smell, but having said that neither is there one harshly unpleasant.

When the body produces an abnormal odor it is usually caused by infection. While most types of body scent is considered socially unlikeable, there are several considered benign while others serve as attractants. Most noxious are those created in the intestinal tract, the mouth, on the feet and under the arms.

Intestinal tract gas (flatus) is a usual product of digestion. It occurs when bacteria already resident in the gut process the carbohydrates in food that can't be broken down by digestive enzymes, or from swallowing gas-containing products such as fizzy drinks or taking in too much air.

Types of odor depend on the kinds of bacteria that inhabit the human intestinal tract, and the food sorts you eat. While normally passed through the bottom some gas is missed, and is then released through the mouth. (burping)

Bad breath (halitosis) is normally reasoned by too much bacteria growing on or between the teeth. Plaque, dry mouth and cavities can also be accountable for halitosis.

While saliva's natural antibacterial action cleans the mouth and removes stubborn food particles lodged between the teeth, it is its reduced flow late in the evening that causes morning breath.

Bad breath can also occur from something in the lungs or gastrointestinal tract. Specific foods like curry, onions, spices, garlic, and alcohol can create bad breath after passing through the bloodstream and exhaled by the lungs. Smelly breath is a common concern people seriously worry about.

Bad breath is one of the most common hygiene perennial problem which can be easily cured with proper effective bad breath remedies. If you are one of the women population that has that problem, don't be depressed, I have some recommendations for you.

Let's face it, bad breath it is not something you can just ignore as it puts you in an embarrassing situations in social life, even your friends can sometimes avoid you because of it.

Sometimes you see some women covering their nose when you talk, isn't that just something you need to take care of? For that to happen, there are plenty of bad breath remedies which can bring back fragrance in your mouth.

The first thing you need to do, is that you identify what causes you to have such not good smelling breath, so that it can be easier to apply suitable cures. One of the most common disorder of it, is eating food spiced with onions, or beverages and drinking coffee or fruit juice. Usually, stomach problems also cause not good breath.

You can start following a simple home bad breath remedy which is by salt water gargle before you go to sleep. Salt will kill the bacteria that causes smelly breath which eventually can help you with better breath smell.

You also need to chew mint leaves whenever you smell the foul odor from your mouth, that may be a quick working remedy but it will not permanently cure your breath.

Another good remedy for your breath is sucking sweet flavored candies or chewing gums, this are considered one of the most effective and simple ways you can start applying. chewing gums and sweet flavored candies are cheap, so you can start sucking them after each meal or snack.

CHAPTER 5

VAGINA

It is clear that because you are here you may have a vaginal odor that is bothering you, or heaven forbid someone else. Normally as a rule a genital smell should not affect them around you, however if it does then the vaginal odor needs to be checked out by your GP.

We are all aware that the smell of "pubic hair cling on stale pee" is unpleasant, but if you know your genitals are thoroughly clean and the smell "not" like urine, then the cause may need medication instead of warm water and soap.

Yes girls it`s an embarrassing problem, I agree, and because I too am a girl understand your reason for rosy cheeks, nonetheless it is a health issue and needs treating. Go along to your local clinic and face up to your problem, or better still have your doctor face up to it instead.

We women were born and blessed with a lot of things in life connected to our bodies all of which seen as natural, but sadly some of life`s natural`s just is not fair. Natural means acceptance where we have no choice, but nevertheless we have the unnatural, which means something is not right and needs correcting.

Vaginal odors are natural, but depending on the strength and of what the actual smell is about, is all the more reason to suspect the unnatural. Although the vagina itself is an odorless organ, every woman has a vaginal odor brought about by something or other, so we accept this; however what we do not have to accept is the unpleasantness of a specific odor.

You have to look after the vagina in respect of cleanliness. Poor hygiene is an issue looked into primarily as to being the cause. Don`t panic this is not insinuating you`re dirty, just a pointer to say that personal hygiene may not be up to the standard required by the genitals to keep smell away.

Because the vagina is an odorless organ it does not generate smells, so if washing the vagina is not done properly then odor can rise. Bacteria at this specific time of poor cleansing, inhabits the vagina, thus resulting in what you believe to be the actual vagina smelling, when it is not.

The following are some causes of vaginal odor:

1.   Bacterial Vaginosis is a vaginal condition that can cause vaginal discharge. This is not dangerous but it can cause disturbing symptoms. The symptoms of BV are vaginal discharge and odor.

Further concerns that might specify the presence of a more serious condition include fever, pelvic pain, new or multiple sexual partners and a history of sexually-transmitted infections.

2.   Chlamydia in Women is a bacterium that causes a disease which is very alike to gonorrhea in the way that it is spread and the symptoms it produces.

3.	Genital Herpes in Women is a viral infection by the herpes simplex virus which is passed on through intimate contact with the mucous-covered linings of the mouth or the vagina or the genital skin.

4.	Gonorrhea in Women is a bacterial infection caused by the organism Neisseria gonorrhea which is transmitted by sexual intercourse. Symptoms of this include burning or common urination, a yellowish vaginal discharge, redness and swelling of the genitals, and a burning or itching of the vaginal area.

Gonorrhea infection in people with conditions causing serious abnormal immune function, such as AIDS, can also be more serious.

5.	Pelvic Inflammatory Disease or PID is a general term that refers to infection of the uterus fallopian tubes plus further reproductive organs.

6.	Sexually Transmitted Disease or most commonly known as STD are infections that can be moved from one person to another in the course of any type of sexual contact.

The only effective approach to prevent STDs is self-discipline.

7.   Vaginitis is a word for some infection or inflammation of the vagina. This is usually cause by itching, irritation or abnormal vaginal discharge.

8.   Vaginal Yeast Infection occurs when new yeast is bringing in into the vaginal area, or when there is an increase in the quantity of yeast already present in the vagina relation to the quantity of normal bacteria.

This is not considered to be a sexually transmitted infection (STD), given that Candida may be present in the normal vagina, and the condition does happen in celibate women.

On the other hand, it is probable for men to build up symptoms of skin irritation of the penis from a yeast infection right after sexual intercourse with an infected partner.

It`s difficult to prevent all bacterium entering the vagina, but nevertheless you can help put a restriction on the amount of which enters. Regular questions like "Why have I got a smelly vagina"or "I wash everyday but my vagina still smells" are perfectly normal queries by worried women.

Well most bacteria, parasites or yeasts inside the vagina will usually generate odors through waste or by product therefore causing characteristic smells. One smell more often asked about the cause of, is, the fishy smell. And the regular answer is nearly always answered back with "bacterial vaginosis."

Bacterial vaginosis is a vaginal infection. Most bad vaginal odors are nearly always connected to infection. A smelly vagina can happen because of many things, and chemicals being one of those. The vagina is self-cleaning so needs nothing more than a little mild soap and warm water to freshen it up.

Particular bathroom toiletries contain chemicals and if in contact with the vulva it can strip it of its natural oils leaving it dry and irritated and also prone to infection (yeast.) Chemicals can potentially slip into the urethra causing urinary tract infections.

Certain chemicals can upset the natural PH of the vagina which causes an overgrowth of anaerobic bacteria, genital mycoplasmas, and gardnerella vaginalis, with reduced or absent lactobacilli. Other signs to say something`s wrong are if there is change in your normal vaginal discharge such as color, smell and consistency.

If bacterial growth unsettles this causes bacterial vaginosis, symptoms of which include a bad 'fishy' smell and excessive discharge. Vaginal pain when peeing (urinating) should always be checked out for fear infection is the cause.

Vaginal thrush is a vaginal infection that brings soreness. Vaginal thrush is a yeast infection; it is an overgrowth of yeast that leads to a range of unpleasant symptoms, such as itching and pain around the vagina.

Thrush can be recurring and it is because of this that it can affect and disrupt a woman`s sexual activities. This yeast is nearly always Candida albicans, but another more resistant yeast, Candida glabrata, can also be the reason for thrush developing.

Men and children aside from women carry yeast in their bodies. This type yeast usually thrives in the intestines, vagina, and around the mouth, but a natural harmless bacterium also in the body, helps keep the yeast levels low. If the yeast unbalances it develops unchecked.

Although the vagina is generally too acidic for yeast to grow wild, it is sensitive to small changes and can easily become an ideal setting for yeast to grow. Too much yeast irritates vaginal tissues which cause thrush symptoms. What to look out for are, vaginal itching, a burning sensation, soreness, and swelling of the vagina/vulva and change in discharge.

Although these are familiar symptoms connected to thrush it does not always indicate that it is. Vaginal thrush bouts can be mild or severe. It commonly irritates the delicate tissue of the vagina and genitals, making it sore, swollen and red.

Bacterial vaginosis is determined by vaginal discharge. It results from an overgrowth of usual bacteria in the vagina, and was once called Gardnerella vaginitis. Bacterial vaginosis is not passed through having sexual intercourse. If you notice change in vaginal discharge i.e. color and amount of loss then you need your GP to evaluate why for these changes.

There is every possibility you have bacterial vaginosis when you experience change as such, and more so if discharge smells fishy. The amount of vaginal discharge considered normal varies in each woman.

It is up to your doctor to decide what degree of vaginal discharge is normal or abnormal for each woman. Aside from smell, discharge from this infection normally shows as greyish white and watery.

Discuss treatment options with your doctor. If you have BV, then your GP may prescribe antibiotics (metronidazole "flagyl", clindamycin or tinidazole pills) for 7 days. Or you can use a vaginal cream (metrogel) or (cleocin.) Be careful when using unknown products.

CHAPTER 6

BACK OF THE EAR

Growing up I am sure we all heard the saying, whether from our moms or on TV, "don't forget to wash behind your ears". Personally, I don't remember mom speaking out those words, but I do remember my dad telling me not to forget to wash some other parts which I won't discuss at the moment, but of course equally as important.

Did you ever rub your finger behind your ear and accidentally smelled your finger and noticed an unpleasant smell, the odor behind your ears is due to oil-producing glands.

These glands produce an oily fat called sebum. The body produces sebum naturally.

Sebum in itself is odorless but its bacterial disintegration produces a smell. These odors are most prominent in oily areas of the skin like the face, behind the ears, under the arms, around the nipples and at the groin.

These are all natural odors the human body produces without will. We can mask these smells with perfumes and soaps, but that's all we're able to do, only mask them.

The odors still exist under all that perfume. For lack of a better description, this is the scent bloodhounds follow when chasing someone in the woods. Not our perfume, but our natural body scent.

Because of the fold between the ear and the skull the oil produced by the gland gather and are not evaporated easily as on other parts of our skin. These produces the odor. But also, more bacteria can collect in between the skull and ear, thus causing a more profound smell.

We have all seen on TV and movies where they rub cologne behind the ears. Well this is not such a wise idea. The oils and bacteria along with the perfume can change the chemistry and produce a smell worse than the original natural odor.

Some of us sweat more than other and most of us just wipe down our faces and forget to wipe behind the ears. Frequent sweating can logically increase bacteria behind the ears and thus increasing the smell. Women who wear glass also tend to sweat more in this area.

For people who tend to sweat more than others, especially in the hot summer season, it may be good practice to carry wet naps to clean behind the ears as needed. These naps also contain antibacterial ingredients.

There are of course many other conditions that can occur behind the ears that are more serious and in themselves cause odors. But these are usually outstanding to the touch and also visible.

Conditions like lumps and cysts under the earlobe. These are usually treated by dermatologist by draining out the fatty oils accumulated. Some never return again. Sometimes the cysts come and go without intervention.

As far as the issue of just a foul smell behind the ears without other serious condition, don't lose any sleep over it. Just good old personal hygiene is all you really need to treat this condition. That is why if you keep your skin clean of bacteria with anti-bacterial soaps, you can avoid body odor.

CHAPTER 7

You've tried several remedies but nothing seems to be working. The rash under your breasts, a candida infection, is causing you pain and discomfort. Each time you move to the left, right, up or down, your breasts shift and the rubbing of your breasts is causing you pain. Wearing a bra causes an agony you never imagined it could.

As a woman, I empathize. Women with large breasts have deeper folds beneath them, giving moisture an opportunity to accumulate. This is unfortunately an ideal environment for the candida fungus to thrive. The good news is there are several home remedies to try that can bring you a great deal of comfort.

Coconut oil. Taken internally it does wonders for internal yeast infections. Topically, it is a great relief to the skin. Coconut oil has a miraculous property: it dissolves the cell walls of bacteria and fungus. Candida is a fungus, and chances are if you have open, inflamed sores under your breasts, you probably have bacteria hanging out there too.

Dissolving the cell walls of bacteria and yeast means that these pests are doomed to die, giving you some relief in a few hours, and a more rapid healing process over the coming week.

Tea tree oil. Tea tree oil also has powerful anti-fungal and anti-bacterial properties. It also has a refreshing, earthy fragrance. Before applying to the skin, make sure you place it in a carrier oil to dilute. You never want to apply essential oil directly to the skin or an open wound.

This is because essential oil is so refined, it absorbs quickly into the bloodstream. When using essential oil, use about three drops for every ounce of carrier oil.

Oregano oil. Oregano oil is another powerful agent for knocking out pesky bacteria and fungus. When taken internally, it boosts the immune system and makes a great home remedy for the common cold. If you purchase as an essential oil, show caution: oregano oil really stings if you do not dilute it.

Since it is so strong, I recommend starting with one drop of oregano oil per two ounces of carrier oil. Do not take the essential oil internally - there are food grade drops and capsules available at natural foods stores.

Garlic oil. Notice a theme here? If you use oregano and garlic oil, you will begin to smell like pizza or a pasta dish. Depending on how comfortable you are with this idea, you may want to apply the garlic oil before you sleep, then wash it off in the morning during your shower.

Garlic oil is also available online or in a natural foods store. Some people do rub cloves under their breasts as well, but I find that this stings quite a bit. However, using garlic oil (diluted if it is an essential oil) has a more tingling, calming effect.

CHAPTER 8

There is a common misconception about body odor, most people assume that the sweat in our body causes body odor which is totally wrong. The sweat that is produced by our body is totally odorless. It's only when it mixes with the skin and hair cells present in the armpits, that it will start obtaining a particular smell that differs from person to person.

There is bacteria present under the armpits that keep releasing chemicals that will then mix with the sweat and cause it to give an offensive smell. In some women, the odor can be quite mild while in other people it can be very offensive.

If you access the number of women who suffer from armpit odor, you will notice that a higher number of women suffer from armpit odor.

Sweating is an important function of the human body that is needed by it so that the overall temperature is maintained. It's very important to keep the growth of bacteria under the armpits and other parts of the body including the feet under control.

In fact we should try to totally eliminate these bacteria on a regular basis. You might not be able to smell your armpit odor as your brain may be processing this smell away from your nose. But that doesn't mean others cannot smell it. Once you are aware that you have strong armpit odor problem, you need to tackle it in the right manner.

There are many ways to eliminate the bacteria present under your armpits - here are some ways to make armpit odor disappear from your body:

You need to shower after any vigorous activity - armpit odor turns to be very strong after any form of exercise or vigorous activity. So, if you are dealing in such activities, make it a point to take a shower immediately so that you are not giving the bacteria in your body a chance to grow and multiply so that they can release the harmful chemicals in your body.

Use good deodorants - even if you are maintaining good hygiene, you should use some good deodorants, these deodorants can be very handy in controlling the bacteria present in your body, and thus you will be keep armpit odor far away from your body.

There are a large number of deodorants in the market - choose the ones that have ingredients that will not cause any harm to your skin.

Change your clothes regularly - you need to ensure that you always have a fresh set of underwear, socks and other inner wear whenever you need them. Avoid wearing clothes that have been used by you previously. They will contain bacteria in them and will accelerate the spread of body odor.

Choose cotton wear - cotton is the best material when you need to keep sweat under control as it absorbs the sweat from your body. That will also help in reducing armpit odor in your body.

CHAPTER 8

FEET

Smelly feet can really affect a person's self-esteem and confidence. Nobody likes to stand out in a crowd especially if feet are the culprit behind the reason.

Smelly feet are mainly caused by perspiration aka "sweat" mixing with the millions of bacteria that reside within our shoes and socks. This sweat is also accompanied by dead skin cells that provide protein and an ample food supply for bacteria to multiply rapidly.

Take into consideration that physically our feet and hands contain the highest percentage of sweat glands vs. any other part of our bodies which helps create this perfect environment for a smell factory much to our chagrin.

To begin the battle with foot odor you must strike back at the bacteria that are mainly responsible for creating your smelly feet in the first place. These bacteria are producing a particular type of acid that is essentially causing the unpleasant odor's. The solution is quite simple kill the bacteria and you eliminate the odor.

You might be thinking that your smelly feet go way beyond what other people experience and this can sometimes be explained by certain medical conditions.

Hyperhidrosis primarily affects females and will cause excessive sweating and thus worsen foot odor. Many antidepressant medications can also have the side effect of increased sweating that can magnify your smelly feet.

More often than not, we neglect our feet until the time that we experience pain, discomfort and even reduced mobility. There are many problems that may badly affect our feet, which include fungal infections, cracked skin, foot odor, corns, fallen arches, and damaged bones, among others.

It is a must to deal with these issues since they worsen with age. With a simple daily routine care, we can keep our feet looking and feeling healthy. Some of the ways to care for our feet are as follows:

• Wear socks.

When wearing closed shoes, it is helpful to wear socks for comfort. Our heel has a layer of fat that absorbs a majority of the impact brought about by walking and running. While shoe inserts may help, socks can cushion this. Comfortable socks are all the more important as we grow older because this shock absorbing layer of fat becomes thinner.

Also, socks protect the feet from the shoe to prevent blisters, corns, or calluses. In addition to this, socks that are made from natural fibers like wool or cotton absorb sweat. There are socks made from special wicking materials, which are designed to wick away the moisture from the skin.

• Wash feet.

Washing our feet is very essential for our feet's health. This is often taken for granted as we take a shower. Sweat and dirt get trapped in between toes every time we go in and out of the house.

To make sure that these areas do not become a breeding ground for bacteria that may cause foot odor; we should soap and rinse these areas thoroughly. It is just as important to dry the feet completely to prevent moisture from getting trapped inside. Foot powder can help in keeping the feet dry all the time.

• Moisturize feet.

Health experts always stress the importance of moisturizing the skin and this is especially true when it comes to our feet. This is because they go through a lot of wear and tear that can result in dry and cracked skin.

This can even become worse in warm and humid countries. When a skin moisturizer is applied overnight, your feet will have an extra soft and smooth skin in the morning.

• Wear properly fit shoes.

Wearing the wrong pair of shoes can lead to a lot of foot problems. If they are tight, they can cause pain, ingrown toenails, and swollen toes. On the other hand, with bigger shoes, heels cannot stay in place while walking. This may cause blisters, calluses, and sore heels.

Shoes should also be made of natural materials to allow the feet to breathe. Leather and cotton are ideal in allowing our feet to feel cool and comfortable. It is important to keep in mind that shoes with high heels can be damaging to the bones so it should only be worn occasionally.

• Exercise your feet.

Walking is the best exercise for the feet. This makes them stronger and more flexible.

For those who easily get swollen feet, an arch support can offer help.

Ways to Care for Feet of Individuals with Strong Foot Odor

Feet with strong odor can be embarrassing and uncomfortable. This is a condition known as bromhidrosis, which is caused by bacteria that thrives on the sweat glands of our feet. Though this may not pose a risk to our health, it is important to eliminate the problem.

• Practice proper foot hygiene.

It is not enough to wash our feet and dry it thoroughly between toes; it can help to use a foot powder deodorant to keep it dry, fresh, and smelling clean.

• Use a different pair of shoes.

We should avoid using the same shoes every day to allow them to dry completely.

Bacteria easily grow and multiply in shoes that are slightly damp.

• Wash socks after every use.

We should make it a habit to use new, clean socks and wash the ones we just wore.

• Use a foot deodorant.

A foot deodorant, whether in powder or stick form, can keep your feet dry and fresh smelling.

• Make your own natural home remedy.

Prepare a 1:1 mixture of alcohol and vinegar. Apply this with a medicine dropper to the area between toes. While vinegar gets rid of fungus, the alcohol kills the bacteria.

Whenever possible change your sock twice daily

Wash your feet thoroughly each morning making sure they are 100% dry prior to putting on socks or shoes.

Try applying foot powder or a non-scented baby powder before putting on your socks.

Inspect your feet regularly for any sign of bacterial infection look closely for red patches or extremely dry flaky patches of skin. Between the toes and within the cracks and crevasses underneath each toe are usually more susceptible to infection.

Stick with moisture absorbing materials when it comes to socks. A good pair a cotton sock will work well for this.

Allowing your feet to breath is also key, your footwear should be made of breathable material. Many synthetic leathers for example don't breathe well and will increase sweating through increased heat. Sandals with a plastic type sole can also cause terrible smelly feet so be sure to select a sandal that allows for the best air circulation.

CHAPTER 9

NAVEL

Everyone has a belly button, but just how did it get there and does it do anything for us now? First off you must know that a belly button, also called a naval or umbilicus is simply a scar. Yes that is what I said a scar. It is the place where the umbilical cord was attached to the body during your growth in the womb.

It is interesting to note that the umbilicus in all humans is in the exact same place. It is located on your belly between your third and fourth vertebrae. Depending on just how the cord was cut at birth will define whether you have an innie (a depression) or an outie (a protrusion).

Most women will identify their buttons in these two categories however there are many different sizes, shapes, depths and looks to each one as it is a personal occurrence.

So if the navel has no use other than to identify us and to use as a fashion statement, what do we do when they seem to start misbehaving with odor or drainage?

Of course the first answer is to see your doctor has he would be the one to diagnose the problem. Perhaps you are too embarrassed to go see your doctor? You should learn to get passed that but till then here is some help.

When we think of an umbilicus infection we think of people that have pierced their navels and though this is true in a lot of cases it is not the only infection you can get of your belly button. The navel almost always ends up being a dark and warm, moist and foldy kind of place, a great place for thing like fungus, yeast and bacteria to grow.

The condition of your belly button, dark, warm and moist is why bacteria get in and like it there, so they multiply and fast. The symptoms of this vary from bleeding, redness, itching, a strong odor, a discharge and pain. With fungus and yeast you may get a white discharge, with bacteria you can have yellowish discharge with scabbing.

Things you should do and not do with your belly button:

• Do not explore, pick and scratch at it

• Do not use harsh abrasive things on your belly button like strong antiseptics.

• Do not rub creams and lotions inside of your belly button

• Do shower and wash with a mild soap

• Do use a salty water base to help dry it

• Do dry the area, even to gently using a hair dryer

Remember that this one area of your body was at first your lifeline to your mother, take care of it and if it gives you problems see your doctor as the belly button can be a symptom or a sign of other problems and diseases.

Do not ever think that a discharge or foul smell is ever normal just because you are heavy and think stuff like that happens in your dark moist places.

CHAPTER 10

DANGER OF USING DEODORANTS FOR BODY ODOR

Most women are not aware of why they perspire. Antiperspirants and perfumes have become so much a part of our lives that we rarely think about why we need them or whether we really need them. It may even be more important to find out if they can be harmful to us.

Deodorants and antiperspirants were invented because more and more people began to perspire excessively and develop body odor. It now appears to be the normal thing to do to give the underarms a spray in the morning and forget about this 'smelly nuisance' for the rest of the day.

But sweating is not a nuisance; it is the body's natural way of ridding itself of certain waste products and keeping itself cool. Like the bowels, liver, urinary system and lungs, our sweat glands are also meant to help keep the body clean. Why else would we have them?

To make your body sweat once a day even for a few minutes is a good way to stay healthy. Conversely, clogging up the skin's pores with chemicals (makeup, beauty creams, sun-blocks, antiperspirants, etc.) harms the skin. Trying to prevent the sweat glands from releasing bodily waste is rather like trying to run a car while blocking its exhaust pipe.

Many people today feel that they need chemical products to control their body odor. This is because other eliminative organs, such as the colon, liver, lungs and kidneys, are badly congested, which coerces the body to dump some of the excess toxic waste into the skin.

The chemical products block its excretion of toxins through the skin, which may please the nose, but causes a steady buildup of toxins in the skin and underlying connective tissues; it also increases bacterial development and the risk for skin diseases, even skin cancer.

Body odor is not caused by sweat. Sweat is an odorless fluid consisting of 99 percent water. Normal sweat evaporates from the skin very quickly and leaves no unpleasant odor behind.

A slightly unpleasant smell under the armpits or on the skin occurs only when your body needs to employ bacteria to eliminate excessive sweat that could not be removed by fresh air, usually because of wearing synthetic clothes that do not permit proper aeration.

There can be as many as half a million bacteria occupying a square inch of skin. In addition, when there are excessive amounts of toxins that need to be digested by bacteria, a strong, putrid smell occurs. Destructive microbes naturally produce bad-smelling gases while digesting waste. The odor on the skin may be a sign of constipation accompanied by poor breath.

It also indicates poor performance of liver and kidneys. The body is crying out for help as toxins are 'bursting at the seams'. But instead of reading the body's symptoms as a sign of imbalance and taking care of it, most people merely search for ways to shut down the symptoms. If body odor occurs only occasionally, it may be due to indigestion or chemicals in foods.

To combat the bacteria most people use deodorants, and to tackle the excessive underarm wetness, they apply antiperspirants. Deodorants contain germicides that kill the microbes and, as is the case with most of the brands, a synthetic perfume to mask the smell of the germicide.

The two most common active ingredients in commercial deodorants/antiperspirants are chlorohydrate or aluminum zirconium chlorohydrate. These chemicals react with the protein contained in the sweat and form a gel that partially blocks the sweat glands' ability to excrete liquid.

These chemicals are easily absorbed by the skin. There is increasing evidence that people who suffer from Alzheimer's disease have large amounts of aluminum in their bodies, which may result from the use of deodorants.

Fruits and vegetables naturally synthesize aluminum. This organic, ionic mineral is not only harmless, but also essential for the human body. By contrast, synthetically derived aluminum is highly toxic.

The argument by the industry that aluminum can be found almost everywhere in nature is highly misleading because these two types of aluminum have completely opposite effects on the body.

The same applies, of course, to almost all minerals and trace elements, including gold, silver, lead, and even arsenic. In their ionic, angstrom-size state (processed by plants), these substances are essential for our bodies, but when taken in their inorganic, metallic forms they can lead to serious poisoning and numerous disorders.

Antiperspirants and deodorants are packed with heavy metals and poisonous chemicals. By applying them to your skin they enter the blood and end up accumulating in the liver, kidneys, breast and brain tissue.

These products may not be as damaging to the brain and other parts of the body if all other causes of metal accumulation were excluded. Typically, a person absorbs between 10 and 100 mg of aluminum each day through use of aluminum cookware, antacids, baking soda, and several other sources.

And although the reasons for Alzheimer's disease are ambiguous, research points to aluminum toxicity that may be one of the primary perpetrators.

A natural deodorant stone costs only about $10 and lasts at least two to five years. It works wonderfully and has no nasty side effects. When you check the ingredient list of a deodorant stone, don't get alarmed when you see the word 'alum' written there.

Alum isn't the same thing as aluminum chlorhydrate. Alum is a natural mineral salt, and is unrelated to aluminum chlorohydrate or aluminum zirconium chlorohydrate. The mineral salts in the deodorant stone don't block perspiration, they mainly just cover odor.

How to effectively deal with body odor:

1.   Avoid too many acid-forming foods such animal proteins, fats and starches. The more refined and processed the foods are, the more likely the skin will have to eliminate toxic waste. The digestion of toxins by skin bacteria causes an unpleasant smell of skin.

Meat eaters especially have a tendency to develop bad body odor. Stick to fruits, vegetables, and salads as your main source of alkaline-forming foods. They also work as natural cleansers.

2.   Stop using deodorants and antiperspirants; they only reinforce the problem by blocking off part of your lymphatic system and dispersing the toxins together with the chemicals contained in these products into other parts of your body, including the breasts. This can cause lumps and cancer of the breast!

3.   Wash the afflicted areas in the morning with a natural soap that contains no harmful chemicals and finish off with a splash of cold water on your underarms.

4.   Make sure to wear loose-fitting cotton clothes. Synthetics will prevent your skin from breathing and eliminating toxins.

5.   You may want to make a solution of your most favorite essential oil (one to two drops in an ounce of water; shake well to disperse the oil!) and dab it on your underarms.

6.   I recommend deodorant stones that are made from non-toxic and natural materials such as potassium sulphate and other colloidal minerals. They are pure and harmless and stop bacteria from spreading if applied right after washing. They are available from most health food stores.

Most colognes or perfumes can lead to serious allergies, birth defects, and even cancer. Most fragrances contain phthalates. They are added to plastic to soften it. When absorbed by the skin, they act as the most powerful estrogens ever known. And abnormal estrogen levels cause cancer.

Synthetically produced musk is linked to skin irritation, hormone disruption, and cancer as well. Natural fragrances emitted from aroma oils are beneficial for the body. Synthetic aromas, on the other hand, disrupt hormonal communication, and they accumulate in your body, building up toxicity.

CHAPTER 11

When it comes to personal hygiene, women not only want to look nice, but they also want to smell nice. Unpleasant body odors can make the people around you very uncomfortable so it is important for a woman to make sure she smells as good as she looks at all possible times. Here are a few tips to help you smell nice for work and in other areas of life.

1: Shower Often

While this may seem like it's stating the obvious, remember that women have hormonal odors that can become unpleasant if they are not showered away on a regular basis. Showering is the best thing a woman can do to combat unwanted body odors.

2: Use the Right Deodorant

There are many different deodorant options on the market and women should look through the women's deodorant aisle and see what might work best for them. Some prevent sweating while others hide odors and there are even options that do both. Find the perfect combination of anti-perspirant and deoderant for you.

Choose a scent you like or an unscented option if you are sensitive to the fragrances. Women might want to experiment with a few different types in order to ensure that they have found the brand and product that is most effective for them.

3: Use Perfume, Lightly

Many women enjoy the accentuated scents they can have with perfumes. Perfume is a great way to mask odors and add a pleasant scent, but women should only spritz it on, not cover themselves with it. Spray the perfume lightly on the neck, wrists, and the back of the knees in minute portions to get the best results.

4: Brush Your Teeth Regularly

It is a good idea for women to take a toothbrush and toothpaste along with them in their purses so they can brush their teeth throughout the day. Most dentists recommend brushing first thing in the morning and last thing at night, but if a woman wants to have the freshest breath throughout the day, brushing after every meal is a good idea. If she does not have her toothbrush along at all times, breath mints or gum can help.

5: Avoid Wearing Sweat-Inducing Clothing

If a woman often gets hot, she might want to avoid clothing that is too heavy or tight. This will only make her sweat, which could make her odor unpleasant. When in doubt, it is a good idea for a woman to wear layers so she can take some of them off when she starts to feel warm to avoid activating those sweat glands.

Sometimes, it is hard for a woman to notice her own scent and others may detect a body odor before she does. Adhering to these tips will help avoid unpleasant odors at all times so that every situation is greeted with fresh and comfortable confidence.

CONCLUSION

If a person is diagnosed as having hyperhidrosis then it means they have a problem with profuse sweating in areas like under the arms and the feet. It's uncanny how people assume it is men that have sweaty smelly feet.

This assumption is false, in fact women's feet is just as likely to smell as much as men's if not worse. The body has 3 chief kinds of skin glands, sebaceous glands, eccrine glands, and apocrine glands.

Approximately two million of these eccrine glands release an odorless sweat that consists of 99% pure water along with slight traces of salt and potassium. A particular amount of these apocrine glands which locate under the armpits and the genitals, or anywhere there is body hair produce a viscous substance.

It's a gooey type of substance which affects the hands, cheeks, and scalp also. If it is allowed to settle in a warm environment the sweat will promote further growth of bacteria and fungi. These microorganisms digest components of sweat and discharge volatile chemicals that are responsible for acrid odor.

Women with a specific odor derived from a certain body part may find their smell is different to another person's who's same body part is affected. This is because people differ, and on the stage the problem has been allowed to advance to.

In most cases of women having a fishy odor, it is usually caused by vaginal infection called bacterial vaginosis, however there is also a rare genetic disorder called trimethylaminuria, or fish odor syndrome which brings the fishy stench not only on their breath, but also in their sweat and urine.

As of yet there's still no given reason for why it happens but research states that the condition is the outcome of defects in an enzyme that breaks down trimethyl-amine, a byproduct of protein digestion freed by bacteria in the gut.

The byproduct is the tiny molecule accountable for the nasty odor at low concentrations and a fishy odor in bigger amounts.

An abnormal odor is usually caused by illness and infection but most common of all causes is poor hygiene. If personal care lacks a proper cleansing routine, then what do you expect?

Try this experiment; pour a little milk onto a saucer and leave. Go back after 48 hours and you'll find after taking a whiff it doesn't smell as fresh as it did when you first poured it.

The longer it's left the more rancid the smell. I know you're thinking 48 hours is a long time but you'd be surprised how many people go this length without washing certain parts of their body. A lot of people tend to forget there is more than the face and hands to wash on a daily basis.

Effective ways to treat and prevent body odor

1.   Watch what you eat because it's said you are what you eat. This makes sense when smells your body releases has people turn their back on you. Particularly spicy foods and those containing garlic can increase body odor so avoid these food types if possible.

2.   Leave shoes off at every convenience to allow them to air while giving your feet space to breathe at the same time.

3.   Use medicated soap instead of ordinary. Since body odor is the result of apocrine secretions combined with bacteria, medicated soap can for a short period of time help you rid or keep nasty odors to a minimum.

Be careful with antibacterial soaps because particular sorts are known to dry out and irritate the skin. If your skin is sensitive and prone to drying out then try Dove or Cetaphil to help put back moisture.

4.   It's a sensible move to carry baby wipes if you sweat heavy. They are handy to have. Remember if you're under stress the sweat glands go berserk and secrete more odor-

producing moisture than normal. You could also use pre-moistened towelettes to remove smelly residue instantly.

5.   Socks made from fabric that suffocate the feet will cause foot odor. Make sure material is absorbent. It needs to be able to soak up and absorb moisture. Socks made from a synthetic called polypropylene are your best bet to help prevent smelly feet. To prevent foot odor change socks regular.

6.   Odor-producing bacteria thrive in warm moist places so dust in areas you're prone to sweating heavy with talcum powder. If you suffer from yeast infections then avoid products that contain cornstarch.

If the problem of smelly feet is the result of ingrained fungus you may need advice of the pharmacist or your doctor. Ingrained fungus is most frequently responsible for foot odor and chronic athlete's foot. If you suffer one of these conditions, then most likely you will need something stronger than soap and water to clear the odor.

Medication containing miconazole nitrate found in Desenex spray, or clotrimazole, found in Crux or Mycelex cream is normally powerful enough to destroy the source of the concern and also considered one of the best effective treatments.

Save yourself further embarrassment if your friends are
making up excuses to avoid being with you,

Get rid of that stinking body odor TODAY!